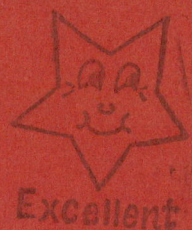

HEART DISEASE

HEART DISEASE

by Mary-Alice
and Marianne Tully

FRANKLIN WATTS
NEW YORK | LONDON | TORONTO | SYDNEY | 1980
A FIRST BOOK

FOR CATHERINE

Photographs courtesy of: Wide World Photos: p. 19; Taurus Photos (by Martin M. Rotker): p. 31; National Institutes of Health, National Heart, Lung, and Blood Institute: pp. 34, 37; American Heart Association: p. 55.

Illustrations courtesy of Vantage Art, Inc.

Library of Congress Cataloging in Publication Data

Tully, Mary-Alice.
    Heart disease.

    (A First book)
    Bibliography: p.
    Includes index.
    SUMMARY: Discusses the history of heart study, the function of the heart, and the symptoms, causes, cures, and prevention of various heart diseases.
    1. Heart—Diseases—Juvenile literature. [1. Heart—Diseases] I. Tully, Marianne, joint author. II. Title.
RC681.T78   616.1'2   80–13712
ISBN 0–531–04163–8

Copyright © 1980 by Mary-Alice and Marianne Tully
All rights reserved
Printed in the United States of America
6 5 4 3 2 1

Contents

Chapter 1
1 INTRODUCTION

Chapter 2
EARLY HISTORY OF
3 HEART STUDY

Chapter 3
9 THE WORK OF THE HEART

Chapter 4
DIAGNOSIS:
15 THE TOOLS OF THE TRADE

Chapter 5
ATHEROSCLEROSIS AND
CORONARY ARTERY DISEASE:
21 CLOGGED TUBES

Chapter 6
28 HEART ATTACKS AND ARRHYTHMIAS

Chapter 7
33 HEART SURGERY: SPARE PARTS

Chapter 8
RHEUMATIC FEVER AND
VALVE DAMAGE:
39 INFECTION STRIKES THE HEART

Chapter 9
BIRTH DEFECTS OF THE HEART:
44 THE MALFORMED HEART

Chapter 10
CONGESTIVE HEART FAILURE:
49 THE EXHAUSTED HEART

Chapter 11
53 HIGH BLOOD PRESSURE

58 Glossary

61 For Further Reading

62 Index

HEART DISEASE

Chapter 1
INTRODUCTION

The moist tissue glistens under the lights of the television camera. A surgeon's knife exposes the arteries, the veins, the fat cushions, the muscle itself of the human heart. We see movement in waves and pulses. The raw life is hard to look at—especially when it is threatened not only by the disease that is damaging the heart, but also by the risk of the operation.

Less than one hundred years ago, surgeons thought that nature had set a limit: the heart was not to be touched. If this rule was not respected, it was thought that instant death would result.

In 1896 Dr. Ludwig Rehn of Germany showed how tough the human heart was. He closed a knife wound of the heart with three stitches. In doing so, he challenged the limit and opened the heart to the wonders of modern surgery. Fantastic repair work can be done on the human heart today. It can even be televised for all to see.

The following chapters will describe the tremendous progress that has been made in our understanding of the heart and its function. We will trace ideas from the dim beginnings in history to the complex understanding of today.

Many things affect the heart, and many things can go wrong with it. We list them all under the label "heart disease." The heart cannot operate by itself. It works with the blood vessels and forms the body's cardiovascular system. The word *cardiovascular* comes from the Greek word *kardia* ("heart") and the Latin word *vasculum* ("small vessel"). We also refer to "cardiovascular" diseases. Cardiovascular diseases affect more than 29 million people and are responsible for about 1 million deaths per year in the United States alone. The nature of these diseases will be described, as well as the symptoms, causes, cures, and prevention.

Chapter 2
EARLY HISTORY OF HEART STUDY

The ancient Chinese, without even knowing correct human anatomy, wrote about the blood's connection to the heart and about its continuous flow. The Egyptians thought that the heart was the seat of intelligence and that it was the central organ of the blood vessels. They knew about the heartbeat and the pulse. But their picture of the total system was wrong. They thought that the blood vessels carried air, urine, and feces.

Erasistratis of Egypt described the veins and arteries about 2,300 years ago. He wrongly thought that the arteries carried air, not blood, through the body. (The word *artery,* in fact, means "air duct.") It is not surprising that the ancients believed that. First, they used the bodies of dead people for study. And when the heart stops beating, in death, the arteries empty out whatever blood is there. Second, as one breathes in, one can feel a sensation of air entering all the tubes of the body.

It wasn't until the second century A.D. that the fact that the arteries held blood was accepted. Galen, a Greek physician, studied the human body indirectly by dissecting the ape. He found that the heart is subject to disease, that muscle makes up the heart, and that arteries hold blood, not air. He was a great scientist, but was mistaken in his ideas about circulation of the blood. Without any evidence, he proposed that the blood passed from the left to right side of the heart directly through tiny pores that we can't see. He also thought that the blood sloshed back-and-forth in the arteries. Doctors after him blindly agreed with Galen, whose work they highly respected, so that the study of the heart was at a standstill for about fifteen hundred years.

CIRCULATION OF THE BLOOD

In the beginning of the seventeenth century, William Harvey set out to discover the true sequence of the flow of the blood through the heart. He did not accept Galen's concept of the pores, or his idea of the ebb and flow of blood.

William Harvey was correct in his guess that valves in the veins keep the blood from flowing backward.

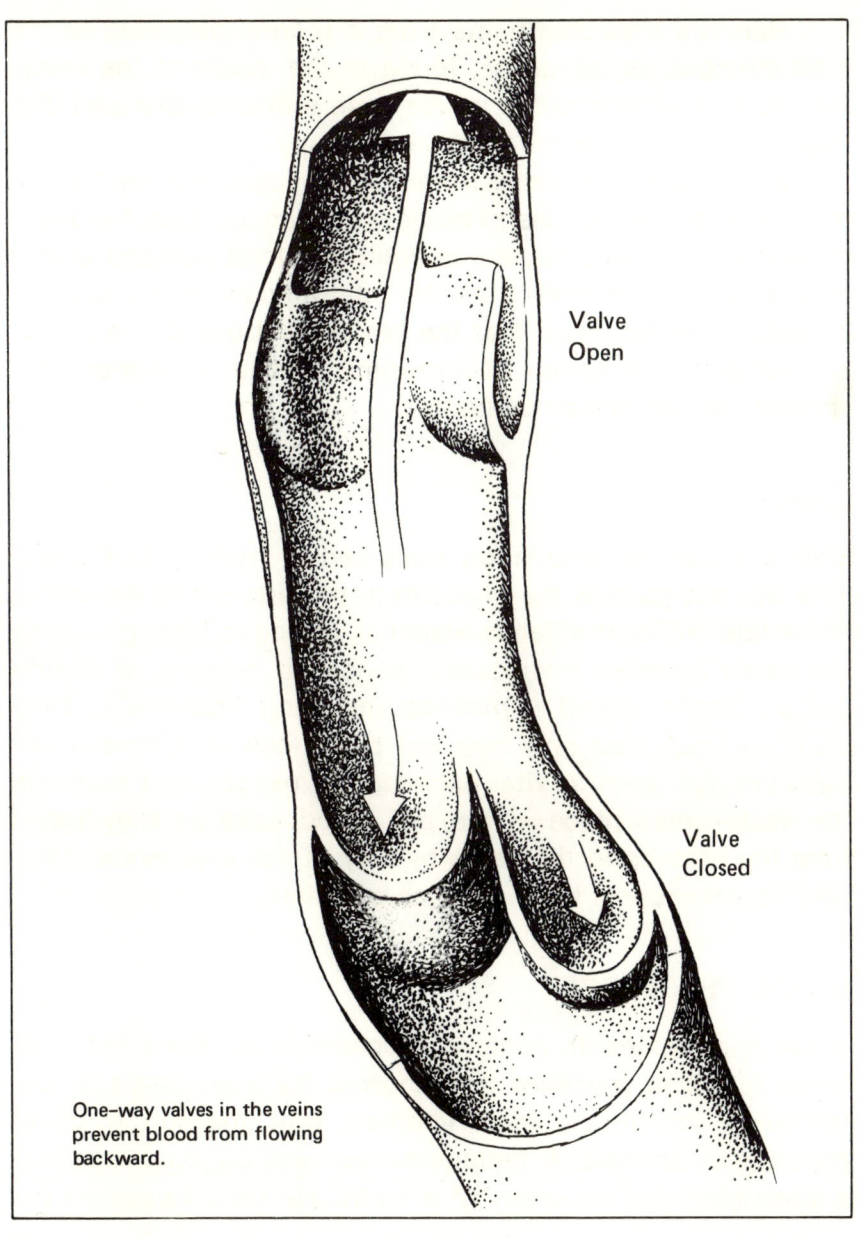

Harvey's first clue came from a recent discovery of the little membranes, or valves, found in the inside of the veins. Harvey wondered why the valves were there. He guessed that they prevented the blood from backing up.

His second clue came from his own logic. Harvey figured that if one or two ounces of blood was pumped from the heart muscle every heartbeat, the quantity of blood pumped in one hour would be far more than the total amount in our system. Therefore, he reasoned that the blood must travel in a circle. He performed a series of experiments and accurately described the path the blood takes.

CAPILLARIES

Only one part of circulation remained a mystery to Harvey. This was the path of the blood from the arteries to the veins. In the late 1600s, the Italian scientist, Marcello Malpighi using the newly invented microscope noticed a network of minute blood vessels, called *capillaries* (meaning "hairlike"). They were so small that only one red blood cell at a time could pass through them. A vital exchange of oxygen and nutrients for waste takes place in the red blood cells as they travel from the arteries to the veins by way of the capillaries. Thus the circular route of the blood was complete.

BLOOD PRESSURE

In the mid-eighteenth century, Stephen Hales found the existence of blood pressure and showed its importance in determining health. He experimented with measuring blood pressure in animals. A famous experiment involved inserting a glass tube into an artery of a horse. He then measured the column of blood, which rose in the tube to a height of 7½ feet (2.3 m).

Hales' glass tube was the primitive forerunner of the modern blood pressure cuff called a *sphygmomanometer*. *Sphygmo* is the Greek word for "pulse," and a *manometer* is a device to measure pressure. The blood pressure cuff was first developed in 1896. With some improvements, it is still used today.

DIGITALIS

Digitalis, the first (and still the most important) medicine used in treating the heart was discovered by William Withering in 1785. It is a good example of how folk medicine has scientific value. In Withering's home town, an old woman used to make an herb tea from foxglove leaves to relieve the swelling of dropsy, a disease marked by abnormal collecting of fluid in body tissues. Withering found that foxglove (one of the plants called, in Latin, *Digitalis*) was the active ingredient in the tea. He didn't know why it was so effective, but observed that foxglove had the effect of slowing the pulse rate of the heart. It is the oldest drug in continuous use in all of medical history.

THE STETHOSCOPE

The French physician René T. H. Laennec improved upon the technique of placing his ear on a patient's chest to listen to the heart. In 1816, he had an overweight woman as one of his patients. Her body was so padded with fat that he had trouble hearing the heartbeat. He needed some way to block out other sounds and to channel the sound to his ear. He therefore rolled up a piece of paper into a tube and held it against her chest, just over her heart. The beating of the heart was much clearer with the tube. Based on this, he fashioned a tube of wood. It was hollow in the middle, flared open at one end, and had an earpiece at the other. He called it the *stethoscope,* meaning "to view the chest."

Toward the end of the nineteenth century, great strides were made in diagnosing various kinds of heart diseases. These developments, along with the beginning of heart surgery, ushered in the modern science of heart study—cardiology.

Chapter 3
THE WORK OF THE HEART

Wanted: Pump to circulate blood through the entire system: must be able to pump at least ten pints each minute; must be absolutely reliable, self-driven and must interconnect with other machines in the system; must function well for long periods with no breaks longer than a half second; must work well under stress. Protected environment and fuel are provided.

Only a strong and special organ could do this job—your heart.

The heart is a hollow muscular organ. It is cone-shaped and about the size of your fist. It lies in the middle of the chest, slightly more to the left than to the right. The heart is divided into four chambers. The two thin-walled upper chambers are called the *atria* (singular: atrium). This word means "entrance halls." The atria receive blood returning to the heart. The two thick-walled lower chambers are called *ventricles*. Ventricle means "little belly." There are walls separating the two atria and the two ventricles. These walls are called *septa*.

The septa divide the heart lengthwise into the left and right side. The right side is responsible for collecting used blood from the body and sending it to the lungs. There the blood picks up oxygen. The left side receives oxygen-rich blood from the lungs and pumps it to the other parts of the body. The heart is often thought of as a double pump. The right side pumps blood through the lungs. This is called *pulmonary circulation*. The left side pumps the blood to the body. This is *systemic circulation*.

CIRCULATION

The blood travels through the body, to and from the heart, by a series of tubes called blood vessels. Large tubes that lead away from the heart and to other organs are the arteries. The arteries divide and subdivide into smaller segments. The smallest arterial branches are called *arterioles*. The arterioles in turn divide into microscopic tubes called capillaries. These vessels have single-cell walls. Through their thin walls, oxygen and nutrients are exchanged for wastes. Capillaries join with small veins called *venules,* which in turn join into larger veins.

The largest artery is the *aorta,* which receives blood from the left ventricle. From the left ventricle, the aorta arches upward over the heart and passes down through the chest and abdomen in front of the spine. The aorta divides into many lesser arteries that conduct blood upward to the arms and head, and downward to the abdominal organs, trunk, and legs. Two very important branches from the aorta are the *coronary arteries.* They curl around the surface of the heart to nourish the heart muscle with blood.

Veins bring the blood back to the heart. Used blood returning from the head and arms joins into a larger vein called the *superior vena cava.* Veins from the lower body join into the *inferior vena cava.* Each vena cava then joins the right atrium. Blood from the right atrium flows into the right ventricle and is pumped out through another large artery called the *pulmonary artery.* This artery branches to the right lung and to the left lung. Each branch continues to divide into arterioles and then into capillaries. In the capillaries the blood picks up oxygen from the lungs. The oxygen-rich blood flows to the venules and then to the veins. Two large veins come from the right lung and two from the left lung into the left atrium. These are called the *pulmonary veins.*

Between the atria and the ventricles and between the ventricles and the arteries are flaps of tissue called *valves.* The valves are like one-way doors. They keep the blood flowing in the right direction. It is the closing of the valves that causes the sound of the heartbeat.

CARDIAC MUSCLE

The walls of the chambers are made of muscle; they contract and relax like other muscle. Heart muscle is called cardiac

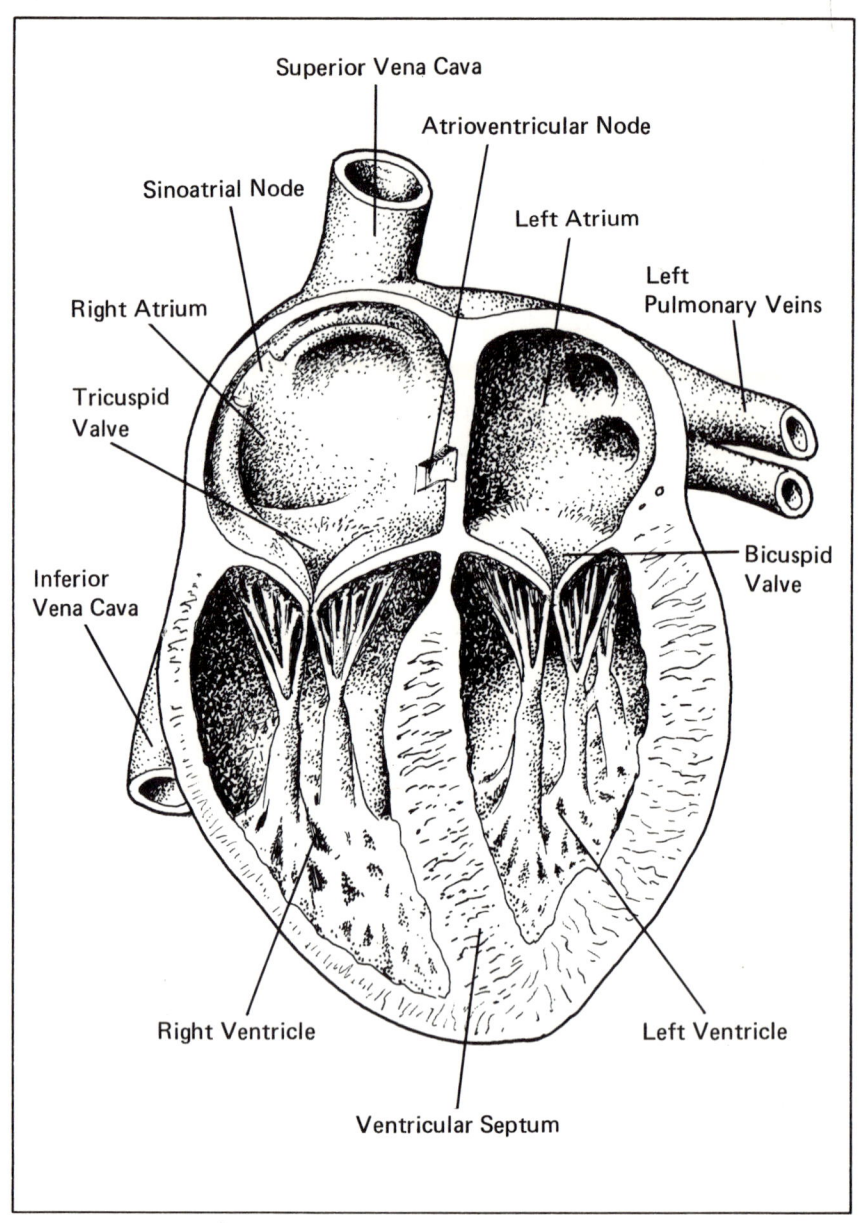

Cutaway View of the Human Heart

muscle. It looks like the skeletal muscles that move the bones of the body, but we are not able to control cardiac muscle as we do skeletal muscle. Another difference is that cardiac muscle does not need long periods of rest between work. This is because wastes do not build up as they do in skeletal muscle.

The thick muscular walls of the ventricles are responsible for the pumping of the blood. The muscle cells are arranged in a spiral and circular fashion. In this way blood is not pushed out, but wrung out of the ventricles. Both ventricles contract at the same time, pumping the same volume to the lungs and to the body. When the ventricles relax, blood from the atria fills the ventricles. When the atria contract, they only pump the small amount of blood remaining in the heart into the ventricles.

THE PACEMAKER

The heart has a special ability to contract and relax in perfect rhythm. Even when a heart is removed from the body and kept in a solution it keeps on beating! This disproved the theory that the heart was paced by the nervous system. In fact, when the cells of an embryo heart are separated, each

*The heart is a muscular organ
divided into four chambers:
the atria, or upper chambers;
and ventricles, or lower chambers.
This cut-away view shows the
rear portion of all four chambers.*

[13

one beats at its own rhythm. Now it is known that the heart contains special cells that make up a pacemaker system. It is this system that sets the pace and rhythm. The nervous system only regulates the pace.

SYSTOLE AND DIASTOLE

The work of the heart can be divided into two parts. The contraction of both atria and then both ventricles is called *systole*. The relaxation of both atria and then both ventricles is called *diastole*. The combination of systole and diastole is the cardiac cycle and is equal to one heartbeat.

"LUBB-DUBB"

The first heart sound, "lubb," is caused by the closure of the valves between the atria and ventricles. The second heart sound, "dubb," is created when the valves between the ventricles and the arteries close. These sounds mark the onset first of systole and then of diastole.

Chapter 4
DIAGNOSIS: THE TOOLS OF THE TRADE

Heart disease is any disorder that interferes with the ability of the heart to meet the needs of the body. Even though there are many different types, there are basic methods of diagnosing all heart disease.

MEDICAL HISTORY

The first step is to find out the person's medical history. The doctor asks about the patient's past health, the health of his or her parents and family, as well as the type of work and living habits of the patient. This information may give the doctor clues about factors that can contribute to heart disease.

The doctor will then ask if the person has any symptoms.

[15

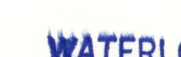

The following are common symptoms which result from heart disease: shortness of breath, chest pain, palpitations (heart throbs), fainting, fatigue, and edema (the collection of fluid in body tissues).

PHYSICAL EXAMINATION

The next step is to do a physical examination. The doctor examines the heart, the circulation and the organs that may be affected by an unhealthy heart. To examine the heart, the doctor taps and feels the chest to determine the position and size of the heart. Feeling the surface of the body above the heart, the doctor can detect certain abnormal vibrations. And most important, the doctor listens to the heart and chest with a stethoscope.

The three sounds to listen for are: (1) heart sounds, (2) heart murmurs, (3) extra sounds from the heart or lungs. These sounds indicate how the valves are working, how the chambers are contracting, and how the blood is flowing through the system.

Examination of the blood's circulation consists of measuring the blood pressure and feeling the strength and rate of the pulse. These measurements give an indication of blood volume, and the condition of the blood vessels.

The doctor will listen to the lungs, feel the liver and spleen, and note the hue and temperature of the skin to find clues. These clues may indicate poor blood flow.

PULSE

The arteries are thick-walled and elastic. The elastic tissue enables the arteries to stand up to the surge of blood with each ventricular contraction. The arterial walls stretch or expand as the heart contracts. They relax when the heart relaxes. This stretching and relaxing causes the arteries to have a throbbing or pulsating movement which we know as the *pulse*. At arteries close to the skin surface, we are able to feel this movement and count the pulse. The pulse tells us the heart rate. The pulse is most often counted from the pulse of the artery that runs over the bones in the wrist. There are many other spots in the body that are easy to count. The easiest arteries to use are arteries that run across bone. The bone pushes out the arteries, making them easy to feel.

BLOOD PRESSURE

Blood pressure is the pressure of the blood against the walls of the vessels. It is an indication of the volume of blood flow, the force of contraction, the condition of the elastic tissue in the arteries, and the expansion or narrowing of the arterioles.

BLOOD AND URINE TESTS

A doctor can also gain valuable information through the results of blood and urine tests. The test results give a good indication of how well the heart and other organs are working. An unhealthy organ can harm the other organs in the body. For example, lung disease can lead to heart disease.

ELECTROCARDIOGRAM —ECG

In 1903 Willem Einthoven, a Dutch physiologist, invented the *electrocardiograph* (ECG). This machine is able to make trac-

[17

ings of electrical signals from the heart. The signals make a normal pattern of waves and peaks on paper. As the heart contracts and relaxes, strong signals can be picked up on the body surface. The abnormal heart, however, may change the pattern of the waves and peaks.

The ECG enables the doctor to diagnose many disturbances of the pacemaker system. It may also show the presence and location of overworked, injured, or dead cardiac muscle. Sometimes an ECG is taken during or after exercise to find out how the heart responds to increased work. This is called a *stress electrocardiogram.* It is used in the diagnosis of coronary artery disease.

X RAYS

X rays are another tool for diagnosing various types of heart disease. They provide information about the size, shape, volume, and location of the heart and blood vessels.

In 1929 Werner Forssmann, a German surgeon, experimented with examining the inside of the heart without open

Louis Washkansky underwent heart transplant surgery in December of 1967 to replace his own defective heart with the heart of a girl fatally injured in a car accident. These electrocardiograms show the irregularity of the old heartbeat and the heartbeat of the transplant.

NEW HEART BEAT   6 a.m. Dec. 5, 1967

OLD HEART BEAT   Oct. 17, 1967

heart surgery. He threaded a small hollow tube, called a *catheter*, through his vein directly into his own heart. This procedure is called *cardiac catheterization* and is a valuable tool of diagnosis. Today, doctors are able to pass catheters through arteries or veins. Once inside the heart, X rays can be taken, dyes can be injected, blood samples can be obtained, pressure can be measured and heart structure can be examined.

ECHOCARDIOGRAM

The *echocardiogram* is a specialized device that sends out ultrasonic waves—sound waves of high frequencies above the range of human hearing—into the body. These waves bounce off the structures of the heart and trace a picture on paper. This provides a picture of the heart walls, chambers, and valves. Their thickness and size can then be determined.

Chapter 5
ATHEROSCLEROSIS AND CORONARY ARTERY DISEASE: CLOGGED TUBES

Coronary artery disease (CAD) is by far the most common and life-threatening disease of the heart. It is the number one killer in North America and Western Europe. Over four million people in the United States had coronary artery disease in 1975.

ATHEROSCLEROSIS

Of all the cases of CAD, 99 percent are caused by *atherosclerosis.* This is a condition in which the blood vessels are narrowed by fat deposits and other cell accumulations along their inside walls, thus causing decreased blood flow. The name comes from two Greek words, *athero,* meaning "por-

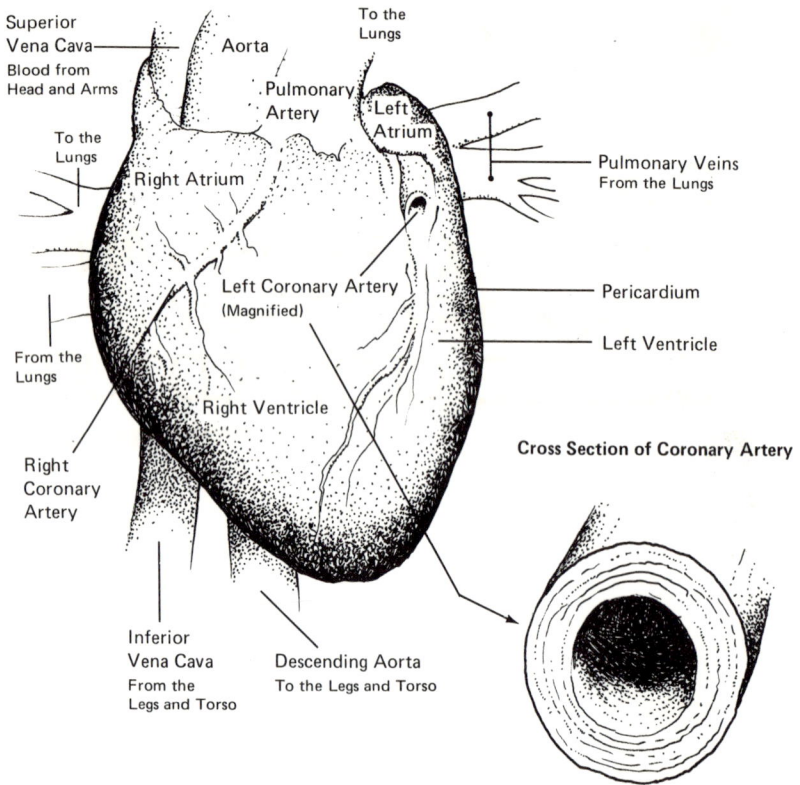

At age 20, the patient's coronary arteries are in good condition.

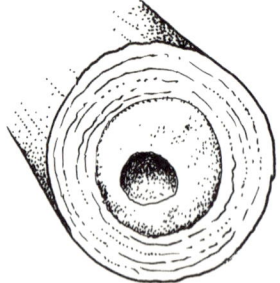

By age 50, fatty deposits have reduced the artery opening to one-fourth its original area.

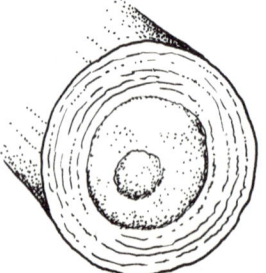

At age 60, the artery is almost closed. A thrombus (blood clot) has lodged in the artery and blocks it. A heart attack results.

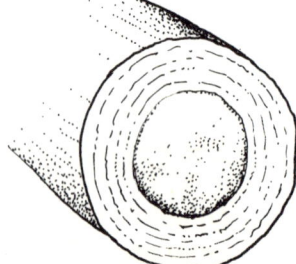

At age 62, the patient has recovered. The artery is completely sealed off. Branches from nearby arteries have taken over its job.

ridge" or "mush," and *scleros,* meaning "hard." The words describe how the fat deposits are soft when first deposited and then harden with age. Atherosclerosis may develop in any blood vessel, but it is particularly serious when it strikes the coronary arteries, slowing down or even stopping the flow of blood.

Atherosclerosis develops in three stages. At first, yellow spots and streaks appear on the inner surface of the artery. Then plaques, white irregular masses, grow out from the arterial wall. They contain an accumulation of smooth muscle cells from the arterial wall, as well as cholesterol and calcium. The plaques take years to develop and there are usually no symptoms in the first two stages. In the third stage, however, there are symptoms. This stage is marked by ulcers, calcium deposits, and clots clogging the arterial passageway.

SYMPTOMS

The most outstanding symptom of CAD is chest pain. Everybody may feel chest pain of some type during one's lifetime, but the pain from CAD is special. It is called *angina pectoris.* Some people describe it as a tight feeling behind the breast bone. But it can also be a heavy or burning feeling and can be felt in the arms, jaws, or back. The pain is caused by an insufficient blood supply to part of the heart muscle. This decreased amount of blood may be enough for the heart muscle cells during normal activity. However, when the body is under increased stress during exercise, strong emotion, exposure to cold, or after a large meal, the heart needs a greater supply of oxygen, which it cannot get. This lack of oxygen stimulates the nerve endings—thus, the sensation of pain.

The pain of angina only lasts about five minutes and rest helps to relieve it. Many people take medicine for the pain. The most common medicine used is *nitroglycerin* in the form of small pills dissolved under the tongue. This drug allows the smooth muscle of the coronary artery to relax and expand. The blood flow increases, and the pain of angina goes away.

FACTORS AFFECTING THE INCIDENCE OF CAD

- Al Nevins loved thick, juicy steaks barbecued on his backyard grill, followed by an ice cream sundae for dessert.

    His brother died of a heart attack five years ago. They used to be business partners. Al's business continued to be highly successful, although hectic. It allowed him to pay the mortgage on his suburban home and other bills by the first of each month. He worked long hours at his desk, and came home tense. He sipped martinis as he smoked a cigarette to relax. It seemed amazing to his friends that such a nervous man could still be overweight.

- The children in the library used to love to sit around Julia Dolloway and listen to her read *Charlotte's Web* to them. She was thin and tall and calm. Julia looked young for her forty years. She rode her bicycle everywhere. She grew her own vegetables in her garden and practically lived on them all year. Her ninety-three-year-old grandmother helped her with the canning of tomatoes, pickles, and fruit juices every year.

Al Nevins is the person most likely to have atherosclerotic plaques in his arteries and a possible heart attack in the future. Julia Dolloway may very well live to be as old as her grandmother. Although there is no guarantee, her arteries are probably healthy.

Recent research indicates that there are several causes of coronary artery disease. Of these causes, the most important are high blood pressure (hypertension), smoking, and high serum cholesterol (or other fatty substances in the blood).

HIGH BLOOD PRESSURE

High blood pressure, or hypertension, will be more fully explained in Chapter 11. It is an important cause of CAD in that it seems to speed up the formation of atherosclerotic plaques.

SMOKING

Statistics show that a greater number of people who smoke die from CAD complications than do people who don't smoke.

Irritants from cigarettes enter the blood stream and seem to affect the linings of the arteries. The irritation seems to encourage plaque formation. Smoking also has some effect on serum *cholesterol*. Future research will clarify these effects.

CHOLESTEROL

Cholesterol is a fat-like substance. We all carry it in our blood streams. The body must have it to function properly and to manufacture vital hormones and chemicals. The body gets cholesterol by manufacturing it in the intestines or the liver, or by eating foods containing it. Eggs and butter, for example, are foods rich in cholesterol.

During the past ten years, there has been a great deal of publicity about cholesterol's bad effect on the heart. It is true that cholesterol is a component of the atherosclerotic plaques. However, some people wrongly assume that if they stop eating cholesterol-rich foods, they will not get CAD. There has never been any scientific evidence for that. The amount of cholesterol in the blood is not necessarily related to the cholesterol found in food. Furthermore, to deprive the body of food containing cholesterol could cause it to make that much more.

Today we also hear the words, "polyunsaturated fats" in relation to CAD. One theory states that the polyunsaturated vegetable fats (such as corn oil or safflower oil) tend to reduce cholesterol in the blood. Saturated fats, on the other hand, are the solid fats of animal origin and are found in milk, butter, and meat. They tend to increase the amount of cholesterol in the blood. Many doctors recommend a diet that includes polyunsaturated fats instead of saturated fats in an effort to lessen the hazard of fatty deposits in the blood vessels.

There are other risk factors that affect the incidence of coronary artery disease. There is more of a tendency toward CAD in some families than in others. Diabetics are prone to CAD. The incidence of heart attacks, caused by CAD, increases with age. Men seem to be more prone to CAD than women. These risk factors can't be modified to prevent CAD, but other factors can. These are daily stress, obesity, and lack of regular exercise that can work to a person's disadvantage. One can change one's lifestyle to cut down on stress, stop smoking, treat high blood pressure if necessary, and control one's diet. These changes can lessen the possibility of CAD.

Chapter 6
HEART ATTACKS AND ARRHYTHMIAS

HEART ATTACK

A heart attack causes a severe chest pain that does not go away in a few minutes as the pain of angina does. It is not relieved by rest or nitroglycerin. The reason is that the blood flow has not been simply decreased, but has been completely stopped. It can be blocked in two ways: the fatty deposits of atherosclerosis can either get so thick that they completely clog the vessel, or the deposits can form a rough surface where blood clots can get stuck. The cells that were supplied by the blocked artery are damaged and will die. The damaged area interferes with the heart's ability to work efficiently. The whole heart is weakened and has trouble meeting the demands of the body. The person may perspire, have trouble breathing, feel nauseous, and vomit. The heart may be unable to contract effectively. This complication without medical help often leads to a quick death.

CARDIOPULMONARY RESUSCITATION

Cardiopulmonary resuscitation (CPR) is a first-aid technique that can revive a person whose heart and lungs have stopped working as a result of a heart attack or arrhythmia. Because the brain cells can only stay alive for four to six minutes without oxygen, the process should be started immediately in order to be effective. It is best to have two trained people doing this. One of the rescuers performs mouth-to-mouth (or mouth-to-nose) resuscitation. The other one does closed-chest cardiac massage.

CPR is continued until the patient begins to breath normally. Sometimes this might take up to one hour. Appropriate medical care follows the CPR.

TREATMENT

After having a heart attack, the victim will enter a hospital Coronary Care Unit (CCU) for around-the-clock care. There, special equipment and trained nurses can monitor the patient's heartbeat.

With prompt and proper care, the heart begins to heal. The blood vessels near the damaged area of the heart take over the work of the closed artery. As the heart heals, scar tissue forms around the damaged area. The recovery time varies for each heart attack patient. Some recover faster than others, depending on the extent of injury to the heart muscle.

ARRHYTHMIAS: SHORT CIRCUITS IN THE SYSTEM

The normal heart beats at a carefully regulated 60 to 80 beats per minute in adults at rest. The normal rate in children is higher. Any change in this normal rate or in the normal rhythm of the heart is called an *arrhythmia*. When the heart rate exceeds 100 beats per minute, as it does in exercise, strong emotion, or some illnesses, it is referred to as "rapid rate" or *tachycardia*. A rate below 60 beats per minute becomes "slow rate" or *bradycardia*.

These variations do not represent real disturbances of the heartbeat, although they might be caused by illness elsewhere in the body. They may result, for example, from fever, shock, or anemia.

There are many different types of arrhythmias. Some start in the atria of the heart. Some start in the pacemaker system itself, while others start in the ventricles. Arrhythmias are serious when the ventricles beat in a rapid and dis-

The artificial pacemaker is a device used to regulate the heartbeat in patients so that blood will flow continuously throughout the body.

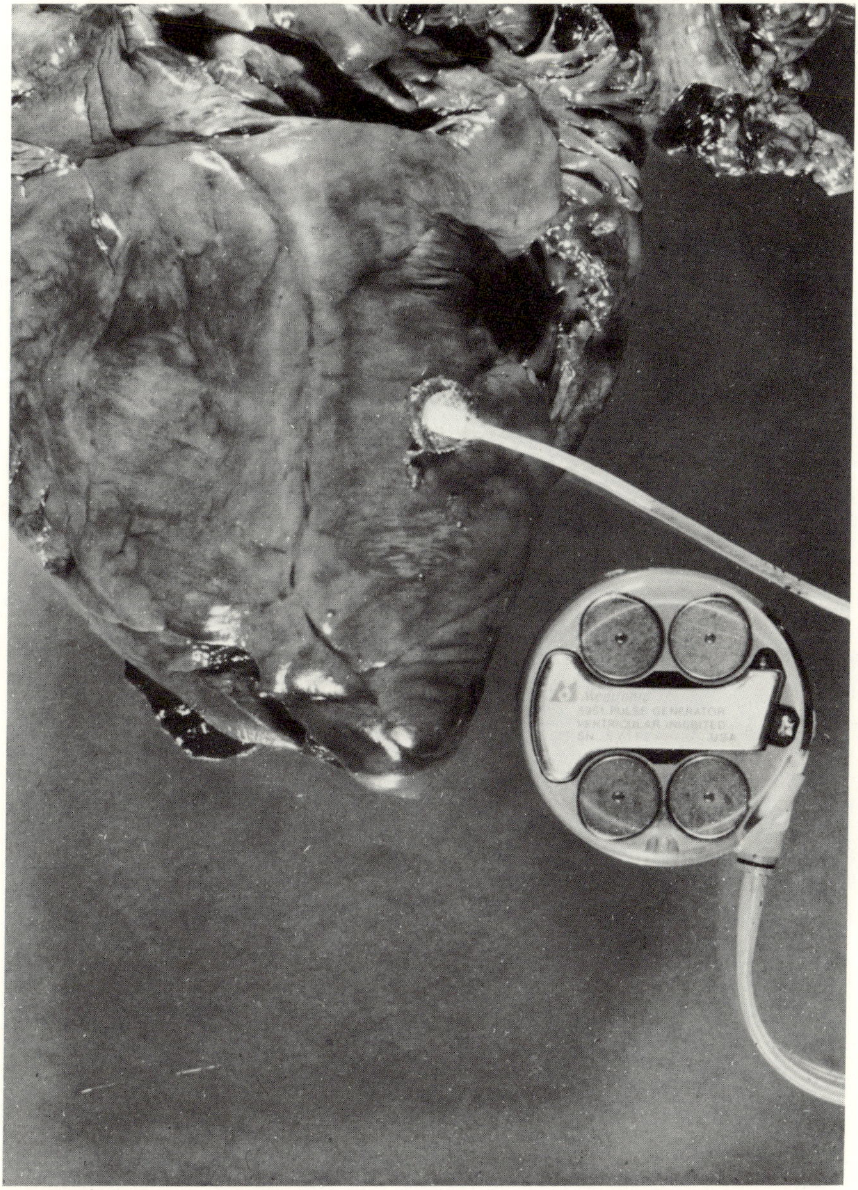

organized way. This irregularity makes the pumping of blood impossible. This is the immediate cause of death in a heart attack.

ARTIFICIAL PACEMAKERS

In some more serious kinds of arrhythmias an artificial pacemaker is ordered for either temporary or for permanent use. An artificial pacemaker is an electronic device that is used to initiate and regulate the heartbeat. Electrodes, placed either inside or outside the heart wall, start the impulse to the conduction system of the heart.

Chapter 7
HEART SURGERY: SPARE PARTS

THE HEART-LUNG MACHINE

The stopping of the heart for more than six minutes causes the death of the brain cells. Historically, those six minutes were the last obstacle to operating effectively on the heart under open vision. Surgeons had two main problems: one, to slow or halt circulation; and two, to detour the blood that would normally enter the heart through a machine that would oxygenate the blood and send it back to the body. The process of cooling, *hypothermia,* solved the first problem by lowering the metabolic needs of the cells. The heart-lung machine solved the second problem for operations of long dura-

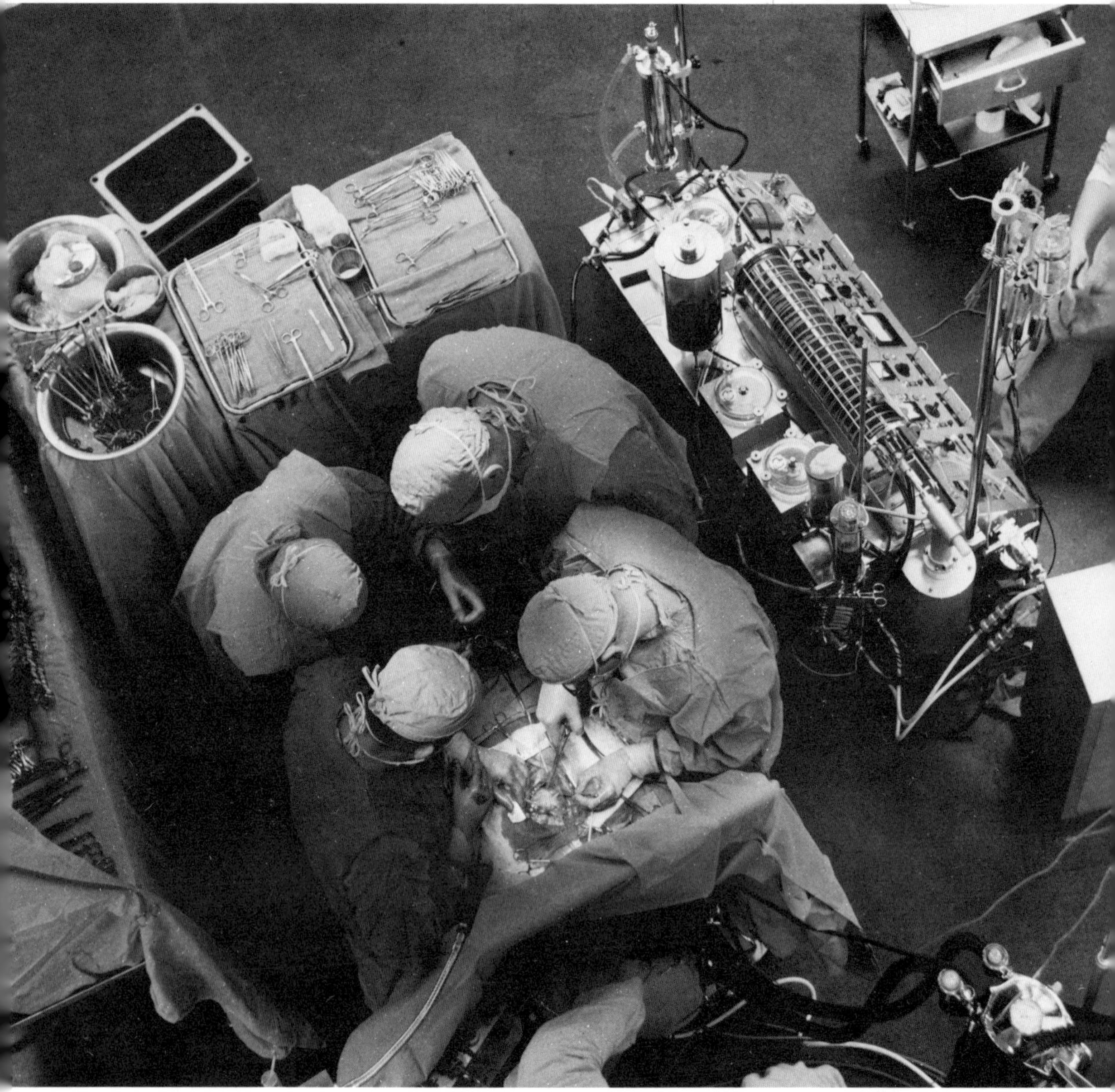

tion. The heart-lung machine is routinely used throughout the world for open heart surgery.

CORONARY BYPASS SURGERY

While the heart-lung machine takes over the work of the heart, surgeons are able to perform any number of heart operations.

One of the most common operations is the coronary bypass. It is an attempt to unblock a diseased section of the coronary artery. There are two kinds of bypasses. The most common is the *leg-vein graft*. A length is taken from the long vein in the leg and is transplanted in the chest. One end is attached to the aorta. The other end is grafted to the diseased coronary artery downstream from the obstruction. Most patients require two or three grafts.

The less common bypass operation is the *mammary artery graft*. The mammary artery is a small artery that runs alongside the breastbone. In this operation, it is divided and its upper end is turned inward toward the heart and attached.

Dramatic progress has been made in recent years in the refinement of open heart surgery. Doctors today are able to repair or replace heart valves, sew up abnormal openings inside the heart, or even rearrange the interior of a deformed heart.

This surgery has been successful in restoring blood flow and relieving the pain of angina pectoris.

HEART TRANSPLANTS

The first successful transplant of a whole heart from one person to another was performed by a surgical team headed by Christiaan Barnard of South Africa, in 1967. Over 400 heart transplants have been performed since then. People who have received the new heart in place of their old diseased heart respond with an immediate renewal of health and vitality. But most of them soon feel sick again and the new heart inside them dies. This sometimes takes a short time and other times a few years.

    The main problem with transplants is not in the way the new heart is attached to the body, but in the rejection process. The *immune system* of the patient's body rejects the new heart. This process is still poorly understood. We know, however, that two things happen: (1) plasma cells attack donor cells and destroy them, and (2) the patient forms antibodies

Although not a reality yet, scientists are hoping that malfunctioning hearts might one day be replaced with artificial hearts like the one shown here. This electric model is powered by a battery-pack implanted in the patient's abdomen.

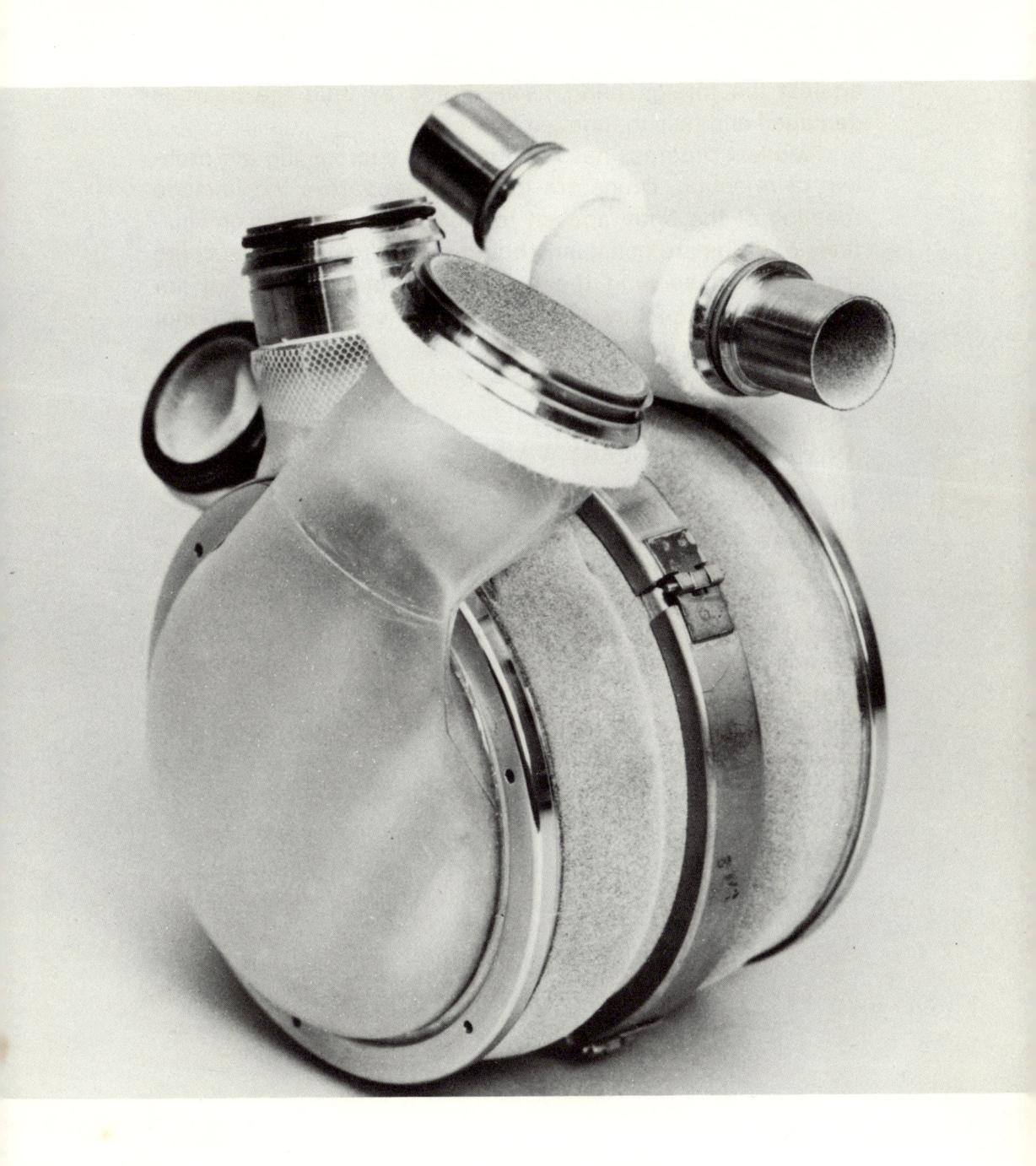

against the foreign heart tissue. Little by little the heart is damaged and fails to function.

Modest progress has been made in overcoming the problem of rejection. Drugs are given that suppress the immune reaction of the body against foreign tissue. Better combinations of drugs are constantly being worked out. Work is being done also in keeping the heart alive outside the body for longer periods of time. This would make many more donor hearts available for transplanting.

ASSISTING HEARTS AND ARTIFICIAL HEARTS

The diseased heart might need help in pumping the blood. Surgeons sometimes install mechanical pumps. Such pumps are called assisting hearts or artificial hearts.

A heart-lung machine is an assisting heart that can be used if the failing heart needs only a few hours to recover. For periods up to a week a balloon type of pump may be installed in the aorta.

Various kinds of complete artificial hearts have been tried out in animals. When perfected, artificial hearts may replace faulty human hearts permanently and completely.

Chapter 8
RHEUMATIC FEVER AND VALVE DAMAGE: INFECTION STRIKES THE HEART

The heart, like other organs, can become infected and inflamed. The heart has a great ability to work during these serious conditions. Most hearts are able to return to complete health without any complication. But sometimes the infection can lead to longstanding (chronic) heart disease.

The heart is made of three layers of tissue that are enclosed in a sac called the *pericardium.* One layer is the outer surface of the heart. This layer is called the *epicardium.* The muscular tissue of the heart is the *myocardium.* The inner lining of the heart chambers and of the valves is called the *endocardium.* All three layers of the heart can become inflamed from bacterial or viral infections or rheumatic fever.

[39

THE MAJOR VALVES OF THE HEART

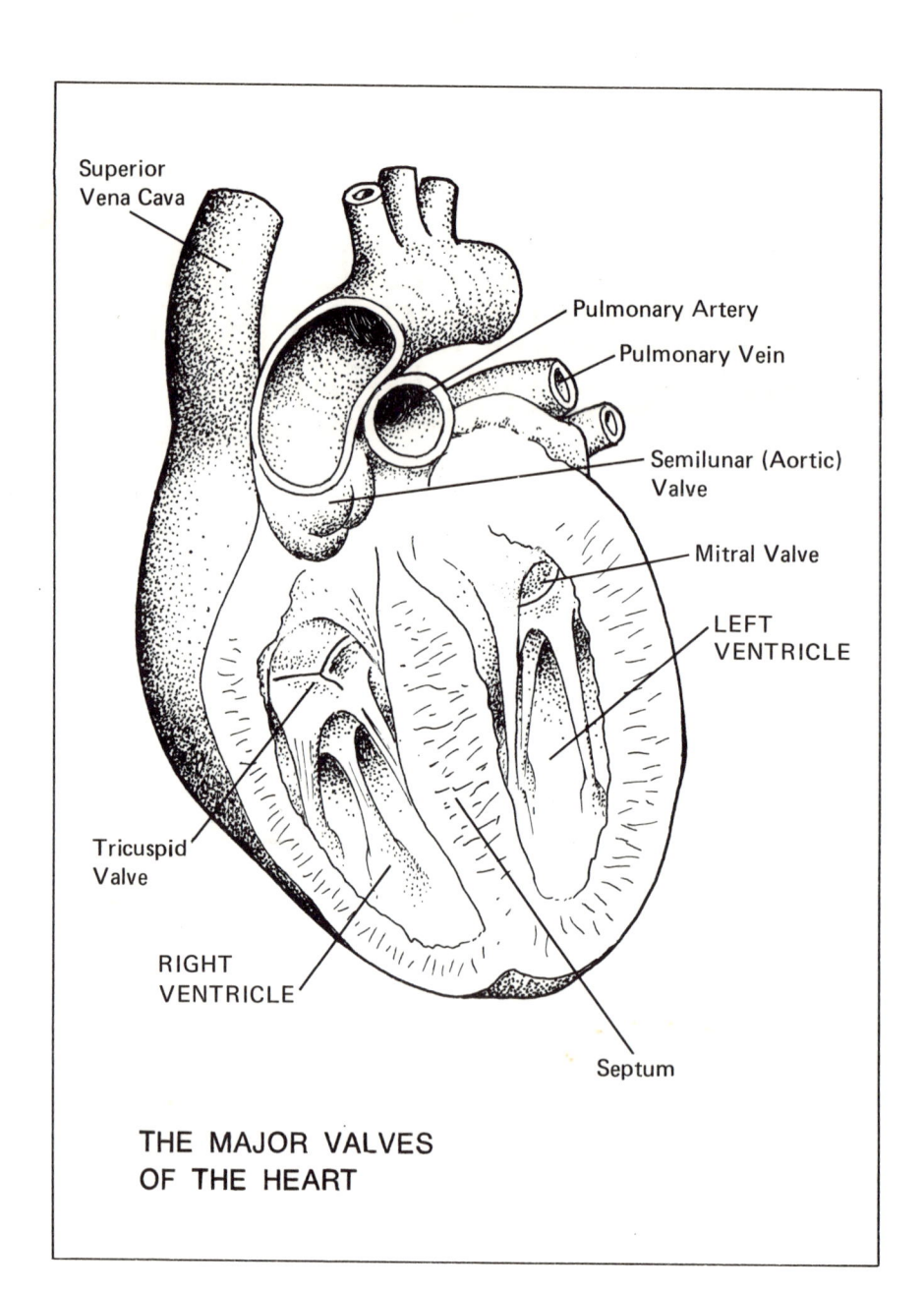

RHEUMATIC FEVER

Rheumatic fever is one of the most important causes of chronic heart disease. It is an illness thought to be an abnormal immune response to the organism that causes strep throat infection. People may develop rheumatic fever after a strep infection. It is estimated that one out of fifty people who have a strep infection will develop rheumatic fever.

Rheumatic fever can involve many tissues and organs. The illness can cause painful swelling of the joints, skin rash, pneumonia, jerking movements, and inflammation of the heart. The most typical course involves the joints and the heart. Tiny groups of cells called *rheumatic nodules* are found in the inflamed tissue. When rheumatic fever involves the heart, the rheumatic nodules can involve the valves of the heart. As the heart heals, scar tissue forms and causes damage to the valves.

VALVE DISEASE

Each of the four cardiac valves can become damaged in two ways: either they are unable to open fully; or they can shorten and don't close completely. When they don't open properly, the heart must work harder to pump the blood past the valves. When valves leak, they are not able to do their job of directing the flow of blood. After blood is pumped forward, some leaks backward. Leaky valve disease is called *valve insufficiency*—the valve is not sufficient to keep the flow of blood in one direction. Obstructive valve disease is called *valve stenosis.*

The valve between the left atrium and ventricle is most often involved in valve stenosis. The name of this valve is the *mitral valve.* Mitral stenosis is almost always caused by rheumatic fever.

MITRAL STENOSIS

The mitral valve is made of two flaps of tissue which open and close. It is wide open when the left ventricle is relaxed, allowing blood to flow freely from the left atrium. After rheumatic fever, however, scar tissue sticks the edges of the two flaps together. The stuck or stenosed valve can open only slightly. The amount of trouble a stenosed valve causes depends on how small the valve opening is. An opening of one half the normal size does not cause problems. Problems begin when the hole is one third or less than the original opening.

Since blood cannot flow freely into the ventricle, pressure builds in the left atrium. The increased pressure causes the muscle cells of the atrium to dilate and to undergo *hypertrophy.* (Hypertrophy is an abnormal increase in size of cells. The number of cells do not increase, just their size.) This type of growth always means the heart is overworked. An overworked heart may fail.

SYMPTOMS

Symptoms of mitral stenosis may show slowly or suddenly. The first symptoms may be fatigue, shortness of breath, and a cough. A loud heart sound and a rumbling murmur can be heard.

The dilated atrium can prevent the heart from pumping normally. Clots can form, since the blood cannot move swiftly through the heart. These clots may then lodge in other organs and cause damage. A moving clot is called an *embolus.* The increased pressure in the lungs may cause vessels to burst, and the person may cough up blood.

TREATMENT

The first successful operation on mitral stenosis was performed in 1948 by an American surgeon, Charles P. Bailey. He pried the valve flaps apart, using his finger and a special hooked knife.

Valves now can be replaced by artificial valves. This carries a greater risk, since this involves open heart surgery.

PREVENTION

Mitral stenosis is preventable. Since the cause usually is rheumatic fever, and rheumatic fever only occurs after a strep infection, the answer is to prevent strep infections. The public is encouraged to seek medical attention when they have a sore throat and fever. A sore throat sometimes means a strep infection and can be diagnosed by a throat culture. If it is confirmed, it is very important that the patient follow a full course of antibiotic treatment.

Chapter 9
BIRTH DEFECTS OF THE HEART: THE MALFORMED HEART

The heart begins to form before the human embryo is even a month old. At first, the heart is a simple tube about one sixteenth of an inch (1.56 mm) long. The fluid in it moves back and forth. Soon the flow becomes directed in a rhythmic movement from the bottom of the tube (venous end) to the top of the tube (arterial end).

Within a few days the tube becomes folded in upon itself, first in a U-shape and then into an S-shape. The venous end of the tube bulges into a pocket. This is the primitive atrium. The middle section of the S-shaped loop enlarges into a baglike primitive ventricle. The arterial end grows into a single trunk.

At this point, the heart is two-chambered. Development continues, however, as two ridges inside each of the chambers begin to grow and join together into the septa. This is a crucial period of development for the heart.

The next step is the formation of a cushion of cells between the atria and the ventricles. These cells grow into part of the septum between the atria and the ventricles, and into the atrioventricular (A-V) valves.

Finally, the arterial trunk develops a spiral septum within it. This eventually divides the tube into the pulmonary artery and the aorta. At the base of each of these vessels, groups of cells form valves.

At about the second month of life, the heart looks like a tiny replica of the adult heart. It does not yet, however, function as an adult heart. The main difference between fetal circulation and permanent circulation after birth is that the process of oxygenation does not occur in the fetal lungs. They do not yet contain air. Only a small amount of blood needs to flow through the lungs to nourish the cells. The remainder of blood bypasses the lungs.

Another difference between the two-month-old and adult heart is that in fetal circulation the two sides of the heart are not completely separated. They are joined by two channels not present in the adult. After entering the heart through the right atrium and passing through the right ventricle, the fetal blood may be *shunted* (or diverted from its normal path) in one of two directions. Some blood may go to the left ventricle. And much of the blood goes through a tube from the right ventricle directly to the aorta.

The fetal blood is then shunted from the aorta through the *umbilical arteries.* They are long blood vessels that lead out of the fetus' abdomen through the umbilical cord to the *placenta*. The placenta is a mass of blood vessels that are attached to the mother's womb. Through this connection, the fetus draws oxygen from the mother's blood into its own blood. The blood of the fetus is not as rich in oxygen as its mother's. There is not as great a demand for oxygen because the activity of the fetus is so limited.

After birth, the baby must supply its own oxygen. As the lungs expand with air, the blood is drawn into the lungs by way of the pulmonary artery. The two channels not present in the adult heart are no longer used and they gradually close.

Three more changes in the heart take place between infancy and adulthood. One, the heart changes in size. The heart at birth is only 1½ inches (3.8 cm) in diameter and weighs less than 1 ounce (28 g). It grows with the body and is always about the size of the fist. Two, the heart changes in position. In very young children, it lies almost horizontally in the chest. Then, as the chest lengthens, the lower end of the heart shifts downward. In the adult, it is almost vertical. Three, the rate of the heartbeat decreases with age. An infant's heart beats about 120 times a minute. This rate gradually slows down to the average adult rate of 70 times a minute.

ABNORMAL STRUCTURE

Some babies are born with abnormal heart structure caused by something going wrong during the development of the heart. Birth defects of the heart are the most common type of birth defects. They are the major form of heart disease in children under four years of age. It is estimated that seven babies in every 1,000 are born with deformed hearts.

CAUSES OF HEART DEFECTS

The causes of heart defects are unclear. One to two percent of all heart defects are inherited, so heredity is only a small factor. Disturbances in the mother's system during pregnancy seem to be a big factor. These disturbances include infection, poor nutrition, the use of drugs, and low oxygen content of the blood. These factors appear to have an indirect effect on the development of the fetus. One example is the effect of German measles (a viral infection). Women who have German measles during the first two months of pregnancy give birth to a high percentage of babies with birth defects. Another example is that there are more babies born at high altitudes (with lower oxygen content in the air) with heart defects than among the general population.

There are many different types of defects. Some are so serious that life is impossible. The babies are born dead or die within a few days. Others are unimportant and the baby lives a healthy life.

The defects can be in the septa, valves, or blood vessels. All heart defects cause two main problems: (1) shunting of blood directly between the right and left side of the heart or bypassing the lungs and (2) obstruction of blood flow, usually caused by the narrowing of the valve opening.

Birth defects do not always show themselves immediately. Sometimes they are not discovered until the person gets older. The only symptom a person may ever have is a heart murmur.

MURMURS

A murmur is an abnormal sound made by the heart. A trained ear is able to tell where the murmur is coming from and its cause. For example, a small hole in the ventricular septum produces a loud swishing sound. Valve defects and shunts have certain characteristic sounds.

SURGERY

Surgery is the major treatment of heart defects. For some defects, surgery is more than a treatment—it can be a cure. Other surgery repairs defects, so that the work of the heart improves. Then there is surgery that is sometimes done just to prevent more complications. This kind of operation is done when there is a certain combination of shunt defects and obstruction defects. If the volume of shunted blood is large, and it bypasses the lungs, an artificial shunt will be made to reroute the blood back to the lungs.

New developments in cardiac surgery are happening now, but the answer always lies in prevention. Whatever the cause of a birth defect may be, it appears to do its damage during pregnancy. Women are urged to seek early pregnancy care; if the mother stays healthy, the baby will most likely be born healthy.

Chapter 10
CONGESTIVE HEART FAILURE:
THE EXHAUSTED HEART

Congestive heart failure happens when the heart muscle fails to pump sufficient blood to meet the body's needs. Heart failure can occur quickly or it can develop slowly. Quick heart failure is called acute heart failure. The slow process is called chronic failure. Congestive heart failure, which places a strain on the heart or damages the heart muscle, results from heart disease, blood vessel disease, and lung disease.

CARDIAC RESERVE

The ability of the heart to work under stress is called *cardiac reserve*. Stress, such as exercise or emotion, increases the work of the skeletal muscle cells. These cells then use more oxygen and nutrients, so they require a greater flow of blood. Under stress, a healthy heart is able to increase its output by four or five times its output when at rest.

During stress the rest of the body helps the heart meet its demands by efficient use of the blood flow. First, the cells take more oxygen from the blood than they do at rest. Secondly, the arterioles constrict in the organs that are not involved in the hard work. The blood flow is increased to the cells that need it most. For example, during exercise, blood flow is greater to the muscles than it is to the stomach. Thirdly, the skeletal muscle cells work with a little less oxygen than they actually need. This is called *oxygen debt*. These methods enable a healthy heart and body to function under enormous stress.

COMPENSATION

The heart can function normally under periods of enormous stress but not under stress of prolonged duration such as disease. The heart does not give up easily; before admitting failure it will use certain tricks to compensate.

First the heart will beat at a faster rate. More blood will be pumped each minute. Also, the muscle tissue can dilate to increase the volume in the chambers. The dilation will stretch the length of the heart muscle tissue, which will cause a more forceful contraction. Finally, the muscle cells can increase in diameter. The walls of the ventricles become thicker to make stronger contractions. If these three mechanisms succeed in enabling the heart to meet the needs of the body, the heart is in a state of *compensation*.

DECOMPENSATION

When the heart's cardiac output compensation mechanisms are not successful, the heart is in a state of *decompensation.* This is bound to happen since the mechanisms of compensation are not foolproof. If the heart rate becomes too fast, the chambers are not given enough time to refill. The volume of blood ejected each beat is decreased. Secondly, as muscle cells dilate too much, they reach a limit beyond which no further benefit is achieved. Finally, while the muscle cells get larger, the circulation to the muscle cells does not increase. The large cells need more oxygen, but they do not have the supply. This problem will limit the extent to which hypertrophy can compensate for increased load on the heart. When these three mechanisms fail to compensate, symptoms of heart failure will develop.

LEFT- AND RIGHT-SIDED HEART FAILURE

Heart failure can start in either the left side or the right side of the heart. Since the heart and vascular system must work together, failure of the left side will eventually cause failure of the right side.

Left-sided failure results from inadequate performance of the muscle in the left ventricle. The damage can be due to hypertension (high blood pressure), coronary artery disease, or valve disease. When the left side fails, the system backs up and causes lung congestion and increased pressure in the pulmonary artery. The main symptoms of left-sided failure are shortness of breath and fatigue.

Right-sided failure most often results from left-sided failure. The right ventricle becomes overworked from pumping against increased pulmonary artery pressure. Other causes are lung disease and birth defects. When the right side of the heart fails, the blood backs up in the veins causing venous congestion. Venous congestion can affect the kidney and liver.

Kidney congestion causes the body to retain salt. When the body has a high level of salt, fluid is retained. The excess fluid causes a puffy swelling of the tissue below the skin. This swelling is called *edema.* Edema of the ankles is an early sign of right-sided failure. Edema can cause a person to gain as much as 15 pounds (6.7 kg).

Liver congestion can damage the liver, causing pain, swelling, and jaundice (yellowish skin). Congestion of the stomach and intestines can cause loss of appetite, nausea, and bloating.

TREATMENT

The treatment of congestive heart disease is aimed at decreasing cardiac overload and improving the performance of the heart to a state of compensation. Chronic heart failure cannot be cured.

Treatment aimed at decreasing cardiac work includes rest, diet, reduction of salt and water retention, and use of oxygen. Drugs that dilate the blood vessels, and drugs like digitalis are also useful.

Digitalis is used to improve the performance of the heart. This drug slows the heart rate and increases the strength of contraction. Cardiac output is then increased.

Chapter 11
HIGH BLOOD PRESSURE

High blood pressure or *hypertension* is strongly related to heart disease. There are two reasons for this relationship. First, hypertension speeds the process of atherosclerosis which can lead to coronary artery disease. Secondly, hypertension increases the work load of the heart. The heart must pump against the high pressure in the arteries. This leads to left ventricle enlargement which may lead to heart failure.

In more than 90 percent of cases, the cause of hypertension is unknown. This type of high blood pressure is called primary or *essential hypertension.* The cause of hypertension can be found in less than 10 percent of cases. Hypertension with a known cause is called *secondary hypertension.* Kidney disease and nervous system disorders are the leading causes of secondary hypertension.

Often hypertension occurs with old age as the arteries harden and lose their elasticity.

ESSENTIAL HYPERTENSION

Symptoms of essential hypertension develop slowly, and may include headache, dizziness, fatigue, nose bleeds, and blurred vision. Often there are no symptoms until the person becomes ill from complications such as coronary artery disease and congestive heart failure. Many symptoms are due to increased pressure in the small blood vessels. For example, increased pressure in the small blood vessels of the eye causes blurred vision. Other organs seriously affected by hypertension are the brain and kidney.

The blood vessels in the brain may become obstructed by atherosclerosis, or the small blood vessels may burst, causing a stroke. Strokes occur when the blood supply is stopped to areas of the brain, leading to brain damage. Stroke is a serious complication of hypertension.

Prevention and early diagnosis are important in controlling heart disease. A stress electrocardiogram test reveals how the heart responds to increased work. The test is useful in the diagnosis of coronary artery disease.

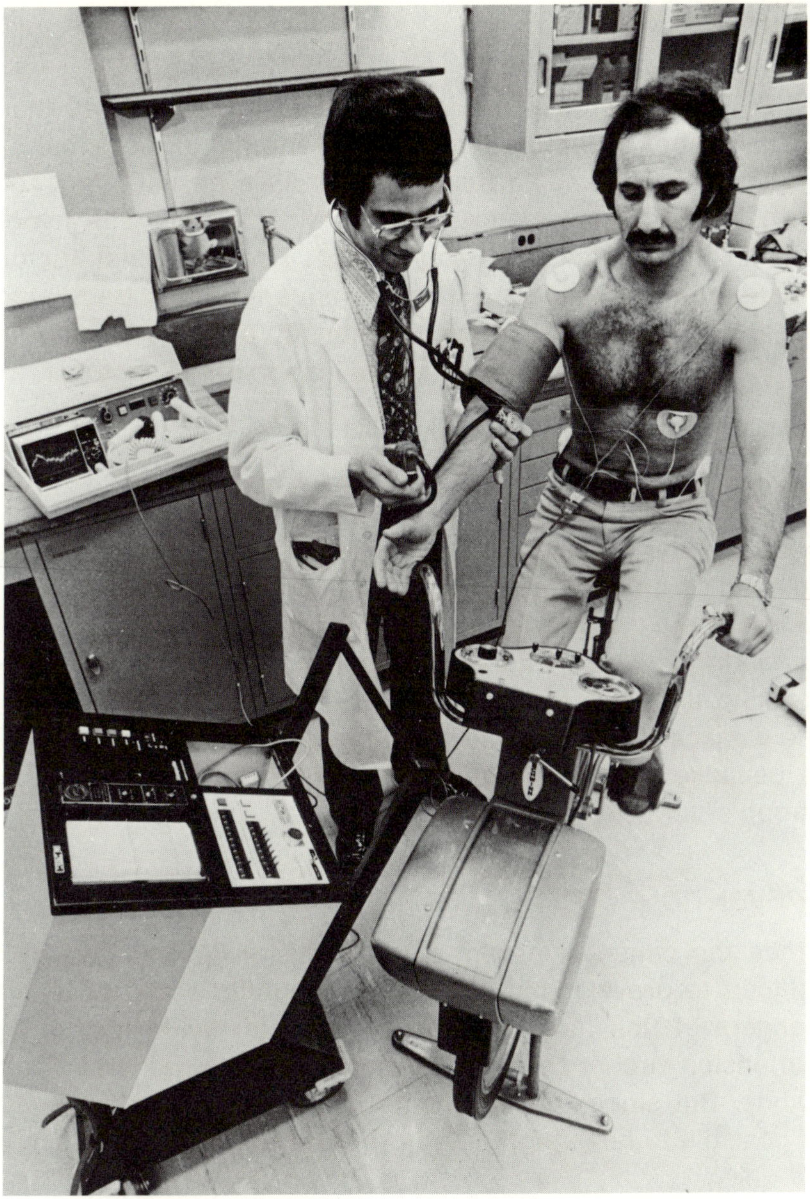

CONTRIBUTING FACTORS

As in atherosclerosis, although the cause is unknown, there are a number of factors that increase the risk of essential hypertension. It is known that heredity plays an important role in the development of this disease. Most people with hypertension have a family history of the disease. Other factors include obesity, emotional stress, frequent urinary tract infections, and high salt intake. Treatment of hypertension includes the use of drugs and the elimination of risk factors.

ANTIHYPERTENSIVE DRUGS

Over the last fifteen years, a variety of drugs have been developed to control hypertension. Medicines that lower blood pressure are called *antihypertensive* (against high blood pressure) drugs. Some of these drugs lower blood pressure by relaxing the walls of the arterioles. The doctor will prescribe the weakest drug that will keep blood pressure normal. This is because weaker drugs have fewer side effects than the strong antihypertensive drugs.

PREVENTION

Since the cause of essential hypertension is unknown, it is difficult to prevent this disease. The public is alerted to the dangers of risk factors. People with a family history of hypertension are encouraged to improve their general health habits. But since the symptoms are not always apparent, it is possible to have high blood pressure and not even know it.

Prevention of the complications of hypertension depends on early diagnosis. The public is encouraged to have yearly physical examinations. Many communities have blood pressure screening clinics. Early discovery and treatment can prevent the serious complications of hypertension.

As we have seen, the heart is subject to all kinds of problems, including atherosclerosis, birth defects, heart attacks, congestive heart failure, and high blood pressure. In spite of all these problems, the heart is tremendously strong. The average heart beats 100,000 times per day, and operates a blood vessel network that could circle the earth four times at the equator. We owe it to our heart to do all that we can to keep it healthy.

And a healthy heart starts with a healthy body.

Glossary

Angina pectoris—temporary chest pain due to the lack of a sufficient oxygen supply to the heart muscle

Aorta—the large artery that carries blood from the left ventricle and distributes it through smaller arteries to the entire body

Arrhythmia—any change in the normal rate or rhythm of the heartbeat

Arterioles—the small branches of the arteries

Artificial pacemaker—an electronic device that is used to initiate and regulate the heartbeat

Atherosclerosis—a condition in which the arteries are narrowed by fat deposits and other cell accumulations along the arteries' inside walls

Atria—the two thin-walled upper chambers of the heart

Capillaries—the network of blood vessels that connect the arteries and veins

Cardiac reserve—the ability of the heart to work under stress

Cardiopulmonary resusitation (CPR)—a first-aid technique that can revive a person whose heart and lungs have stopped working as a result of a heart attack or arrhythmia
Cardiovascular—refers to the heart and the blood vessel system of the body
Cholesterol—a fat-like substance found in animal tissue
Congestive heart failure—the failure of the heart muscle to pump sufficient blood to meet the body's needs
Coronary arteries—the arteries that supply the heart muscle with blood
Diastole—the period of relaxation of both atria and then both ventricles in a heartbeat
Digitalis—a drug used in the treatment of certain types of heart disease
Echocardiograph—a diagnostic method of sending ultrasonic waves into the heart and electronically tracing the way they bounce off the structures of the heart
Edema—the collection of fluid in the body tissues
Electrocardiograph—a machine that makes tracings of electrical signals from the heart
Embolus—a clot (or other substance such as an air bubble, fat, or tumor) moving in the bloodstream
Hypertension—high blood pressure
Hypertrophy—the enlargement of a tissue or organ due to the increase in the size of its cells
Hypothermia—the state of low body temperature
Immune system—all of the organic processes within the body that protect it from infection and foreign substances
Inferior vena cava—the large vein that conducts deoxygenated blood from the lower part of the body to the right atrium of the heart
Mitral stenosis—a narrowing of the mitral valve
Murmur—an abnormal sound made by the heart
Pericardium—a closed sac of tissue surrounding the heart and the roots of the great vessels
Pulmonary artery—the large artery that conducts deoxygenated blood from the left ventricle to the lungs
Pulmonary circulation—the flow of blood from the right ventricle to the lungs and back to the left atrium

Pulse—the throbbing of an artery caused by the contraction and expansion of the heart
Septa—the walls separating the two atria and the two ventricles; the septa divide the heart lengthwise into the right and left side
Stethoscope—an instrument for listening to sounds within the body
Stroke—the stoppage of the blood supply to some part of the brain due to the breaking or blocking of a blood vessel
Superior vena cava—the large vein that conducts the deoxygenated blood from the upper part of the body to the right atrium of the heart
Systemic circulation—flow of blood from the left ventricle to all parts of the body and back again to the heart
Systole—the period of contraction of both atria and then both ventricles in a heartbeat
Valves—the flaps of tissue that keep the blood flowing in one direction
Valve insufficiency—the backward leaking of the blood flow because of a malformation of the valves of the heart
Valve stenosis—a narrowing of the opening of the heart valves thereby obstructing the flow of blood
Ventricles—the two thick-walled lower chambers of the heart
Venules—the smallest branches of the veins

For Further Reading

Meriwether, Louise. *The Heart Man: Dr. Daniel Hale Williams.* New Jersey: Prentice-Hall, 1972.

Silverstein, Alvin and Silverstein, Virginia. *Circulatory Systems: The Rivers Within.* New Jersey: Prentice-Hall, 1969.

———. *Heart Disease.* Chicago: Follett, 1976.

Simon, Seymour. *About Your Heart.* New York: McGraw Hill, 1975.

Simon, Tony. *The Heart Explorers.* New York: Basic Books, 1966.

Weart, Edith Lucie. *The Story of Your Blood.* Coward-McCann, 1960.

Zim, Herbert Spencer. *Blood.* New York: William Morrow & Co., 1968.

For further information, the following organizations publish pamphlets:

American Heart Association
205 East 42 Street
New York, N.Y. 10017

Heart Information Center
National Heart, Lung, and Blood Institute
National Institutes of Health
Bethesda, Md. 20205

Index

Acute heart failure, 49
Angina pectoris, 23–24
Antihypertensive drugs, 56
Aorta, 11
Arrhythmias, 30–32
Arteries, 10–11, 16–17, 45–46
Arterioles, 10
Artificial hearts, 37, 38
Artificial pacemaker, 31, 32
Assisting hearts, 37, 38
Atherosclerosis, 21–23, 28
Atria, 10–14, 45
Atrioventricular valves, 45

Bailey, Charles P., 43

Barnard, Christiaan, 36
Birth defects, 44–48, 52
Blood circulation, 4–6, 10–11, 16, 45–46
Blood pressure, 6–7, 17
  high, 25, 53–57
Blood tests, 17
Bradycardia, 30

Capillaries, 6, 10
Cardiac catheterization, 20
Cardiac muscle, 11–12
Cardiac reserve, 49–50
Cardiopulmonary resuscitation (CPR), 29

Cardiovascular diseases, 2
Cardiovascular system, 2
Catheter, 20
Chest pain, 23–24
Cholesterol, 25–26
Chronic heart failure, 49
Compensation, 50
Congestive heart failure, 49–52
Coronary arteries, 11
Coronary artery disease, 21–27
Coronary bypass surgery, 35–36
Coronary Care Unit (CCU), 29

Decompensation, 51
Diagnosis, 15–20
Diastole, 14
Digitalis, 7, 52

Echocardiogram, 20
Edema, 52
Einthoven, Willem, 17
Electrocardiogram (ECG), 17–18, 19
Embolus, 42
Endocardium, 39
Epicardium, 39
Erasistratis, 3
Essential hypertension, 53, 54

Fetal blood, 45–46
Forssmann, Werner, 18, 20

Galen, 4
German measles, 47

Hales, Stephen, 6–7
Harvey, William, 4–6

Heart
    birth defects of, 44–48, 52
    development of, 44–45
    disease of, see Heart disease
    history of study of, 3–8
    physical description of, 10, 39
    work of, 9–14
Heart attack, 28–30
Heart disease
    coronary artery, 21–27
    diagnosis of, 15–20
    heart attack and, 28–30
    infections, 39–43
    surgery and, 33–38, 48
    symptoms of, 16
Heart failure, 49–52
Heart-lung machine, 33, 35, 38
Heart rate, 13–14, 17, 30–32, 46, 50, 52
Heart sounds, 14, 16
Heart surgery, 33–38, 48
Heart transplants, 36, 38
Heredity, 26, 56
High blood pressure, 25, 53–57
Hypertension, see High blood pressure
Hypertrophy, 42
Hypothemia, 33

Immune system, 36, 38
Infections, 39–43
Inferior vena cava, 11

Laennec, René T. H., 7–8
Left-sided heart failure, 51
Leg-vein graft, 35

[63

Malpichi, Marcello, 6
Mammary artery graft, 35–36
Medical history, 15–16
Mitral stenosis, 42–43
Murmurs, 47–48
Myocardium, 39

Pacemaker, 13–14
    artificial, 31, 32
Pericardium, 39
Personality type, 24–25
Physical examination, 16–20
Placenta, 46
Polyunsaturated fats, 26
Pulmonary artery, 11
Pulmonary circulation, 10
Pulmonary veins, 11
Pulse, 16–17

Rehn, Ludwig, 1–2
Rheumatic fever, 41, 42, 43
Rheumatic nodules, 41
Right-sided heart failure, 51, 52

Saturated fats, 26
Secondary hypertension, 53–54
Septa, 10

Smoking, 25
Sphygmomanometer, 7
Stethoscope, 7–8
Strep infection, 41, 43
Stress, 26–27, 50
Stress electrocardiogram, 18
Strokes, 54
Superior vena cava, 11
Surgery, 33–38, 48
Systemic circulation, 10
Systole, 14

Tachycardia, 30
Transplants, 36, 38

Umbilical arteries, 45–46
Urine tests, 17

Valve stenosis, 41–43
Valves, 5, 6, 40–43, 47, 48
Veins, 10, 11
Venous congestion, 52
Ventricles, 10–14, 45
Venules, 10, 11

X rays, 18, 20

[64

35898